PREGNANCY Questions & Answers

75 Important Questions Asked And Answered

Julie McAllister

PREGNANCY Questions & Answers

Copyright ©2018 by Julie McAllister

ISBN-13: 978-1985667426

ISBN-10: 1985667428

Contents

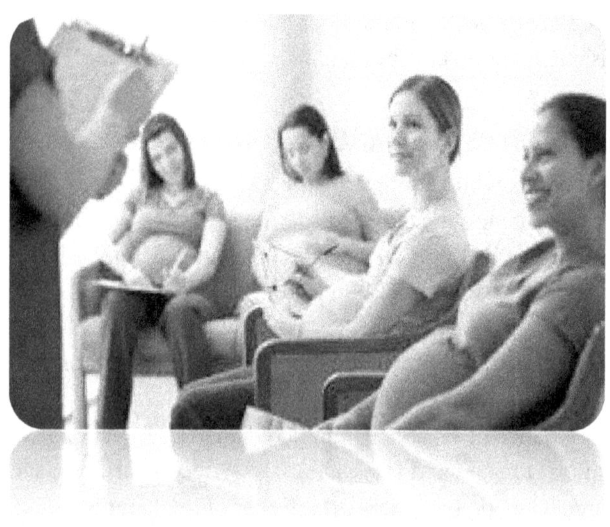

INTRODUCTION

Thank you for purchasing this book it is my sincere hope that it will answer all your questions on pregnancy. For most ladies, pregnancy is a period of extraordinary bliss, energy and reckoning. Pregnancy is a period of physical and enthusiastic change when loads of changes happen normally inside your body. On the off chance that you are a smoker, at that point utilize your pregnancy, or the time when you are arranging pregnancy to stop smoking and stay quit after the child is conceived. Maternal smoking amid pregnancy is related with a higher danger of non-syndromic orofacial clefts in babies. Smoking amid pregnancy is an awful decision. Pregnancy is an opportunity to "tune in" to your body - it is not an opportunity to be abstaining from food, and endeavoring to get more fit.

The way to a sound pregnancy is arranging it in any case. Eating great can enable you to have a sound pregnancy and a solid infant - Healthy mum, sound pregnancy. On the off chance that you attempt to remain as solid as you can amid your pregnancy this will give you the most obvious opportunity with regards to conveying a sound infant at full term.

As a hopeful mother, your best need ought to be adhering to a good diet. Eating admirably should start before you end up plainly pregnant so your body will be supplied up with the supplements you requirement for a solid pregnancy. Not long after discovering that you have considered you should see a specialist, as your specialist can disclose to you about solid pregnancy weight pick up. Remaining sound is doubly critical when you're pregnant.

Exercise is additionally an essential piece of a solid pregnancy, exercise can enable you to come back to your pre-pregnancy weight quicker and furthermore have a speedier, less demanding birth.

Sufficient rest is basic to advance a sound pregnancy. Conversing with a social insurance supplier is a standout amongst the most vital things ladies and families can do to plan for a sound pregnancy. Indeed, even before origination, it is significant to anticipate a solid pregnancy. A sound way of life, even before you end up noticeably pregnant is the most ideal approach to give your child a solid begin. In case you're wanting to end up noticeably pregnant, get ready for a sound pregnancy by dealing with medicinal and dental concerns already. Pregnancy is not an opportunity to be on a get-healthy plan.

CHAPTER 1: WELLBEING CONCERNS

1. HOW DO I KNOW IF I AM READY TO GET PREGNANT?

Thinking about if you are willing or not is a big step. When you are properly prepared, then you will be less stressed about what could or could not happen. Before you get pregnant, it is best that you got to your OB/GYN and got a checkup as well as ask any questions that you may have about childbirth and being pregnant. During this checkup, your doctor will switch you off any medications that you may be on that could harm your fetus when you become pregnant. Moreover, they will also give you the information you need when it comes to folic acid, prenatal vitamins, and everything that you need to have or know about to prepare your body for conception.

2. HOW DO I KNOW WHEN IS THE RIGHT TIME FOR ME TO GET PREGNANT?

The best time for you to get pregnant is when you are ovulating. Ovulation happens typically fourteen days before your next period is set to start (if you are on a regular schedule. This can be difficult to track if your periods are not regular). Most cycles last twenty-four to thirty days, and you will begin to ovulate somewhere between day ten and day sixteen.

3. WHAT ARE THE PROS AND CONS OF GETTING PREGNANT?

Everyone looks at pregnancy differently, so there are going to be different advantages and disadvantages for every woman depending on how they look at being pregnant.

A few cons that are quite common amongst mothers are:

- The decisions that you have to make with regards to getting prenatal screenings, what you are going to do with the results, so on and so forth.

- The lack of alcohol. You are not supposed to drink while you are pregnant. Even though some doctors will tell you that it is okay for you to have a glass or two in moderation, there are others who will tell you to stay away from it altogether. It is up to you on whether or not you heed their warning.

- How pregnancy is going to affect your body.

- Mood swings and lack of sleep. Thanks to some hormones that are flooding your system, you may find that you are more irritable at times than others and that you are having problems sleeping when your baby gets here.

Some pros are:

- Bigger breasts. As you go through your pregnancy, your breasts are going to grow large due to the milk that is being produced in preparation for the nursing process.

- Being spoiled with love and care. Many women experience that their partners, their friends, and their families tend to destroy them when they find out that they are pregnant because everyone is excited for the baby!

- Your hair and nails are going to grow faster thanks to all those hormones (they are not all bad, they just tend to get a little bit irritating when it comes to certain aspects of your pregnancy).

4. WHAT SYMPTOMS ARE NORMAL WHILE I AM PREGNANT?

There are different symptoms that you will experience while you are pregnant. However, some of the symptoms you may experience are:

- Swelling and bloating,

- Acne,

- Cramping,

- Changes in your sleep pattern,

- Sensitivities

5. IS IT NORMAL TO HAVE OTHER DISCHARGE WHILE PREGNANT?

Yes. Not only are your hormones sky-rocketing due to your baby, but you also have extra blood flow going to your pelvis. There is a high possibility that you are going to notice an increase in discharge as you go through your pregnancy.

If you find that your discharge has a colour, odour, is painful, or is watery, you need to contact your doctor right away. It could mean that you have an infection of some sort that needs to be treated, or even that your water has broken.

6. WHAT CAN I EXPECT FROM MY EMOTIONS?

You can expect your emotions to be all over the place thanks to the hormones that you have in your system. You may feel like laughing one minute and crying the next.

7. HOW MUCH IS A BABY GROWING EACH MONTH?

Month one:

It is going to be when your embryo is still starting to develop. There are going to be two layers of cells that are going to help to develop all the organs and vital body parts that your baby is going to need to survive.

Month two:

At this point, your little one is the size of a kidney bean and will be moving. There will be webbed fingers, but you can very distinctly see that he or she has fingers!

Month three:

During this month your baby is going to be around three inches long and is going to have the same weight as a pea pod. Not only that, but his fingerprints have now developed making him his unique person!

Month four:

Your baby is now about 5.5 inches long and weighs somewhere around five ounces. It is during this month that he is going to begin to have his skeleton harden from the cartilage that makes up our skeleton to the bones that are going to help him hold his shape and move around.

Month five:
Ten and a half inches in length, your baby now has eyelids and eyebrows. He is also able to stretch out his legs (this is where you will probably begin to feel more kicks).

The wrinkles on your baby's skin are starting to smooth out as he begins to put on more weight. With that weight gain, your child now weighs around a pound and a half.

Month seven:
Your baby can now see what is around him and can open and close his eyes. Your child is also one and a half inches long.

Month eight:
A baby fills out to be rounder and more fully developed; your baby now weighs around 4.7 pounds. Not only that, but his lungs are now developed and he can breathe better.

Month nine:
You're now ready for your baby to come any day now! Baby is around twenty and a half inches long and weighs about seven and a half pounds (could be larger, could be smaller). However, your baby is fully developed and ready to be held by you!

8. WHY AM I ALWAYS TIRED?

During the early and late stages of your pregnancy, you may realise that you are more tired because your hormones are working overtime to keep up with all the changes that your body is making for both you and the baby.

It is also possible that you are having trouble sleeping at night because of things like having to go pee all the time, heartburn, or even leg cramps.

9. WILL MY FREQUENT URINATION STOP WHILE I AM PREGNANT?

Your constant need to urinate will ease up after your baby is born. In the days immediately following the baby's birth, you may realise that you are urinating more often because your body is attempting to get rid of all the fluids that your body retained while you were pregnant.

10. WHY AM I EXPERIENCING HEADACHES WHILE I AM PREGNANT?

You may be experiencing headaches that range from mild to intense due to the rise in hormone production. This is your body's way of trying to accommodate the sudden increases in hormones. Once your body is used to the hormones, your headache should ease up. If they do not, it is best that you talk to your health care provider.

11. DOES BEING PREGNANT CAUSE LOWER BACK PAIN?

Yes, pregnancy does cause lower back pain. It is usually caused because your centre of gravity has shifted to the front of your body due to your ever-growing abdomen. Changing the way that you sit and can help to ease some of the back pain that you are feeling. If you sleep on your side, you may want to place a pillow between your knees.

You may feel an increase in back pain right before you go into labour.

12. HOW DO I TREAT MORNING SICKNESS?

It's an unpleasant side effect, but your baby is not at increased risk. Most women find it starts to blow over by week 16 to 20. The following may help to reduce the symptoms; sometimes it is a case of trial and error.

- Get plenty of rest: tiredness can increase nausea.

- Ensure you drink plenty of water, to stay hydrated, but sip fluid. Little and often is better than one large drink, you may find you vomit otherwise. Drinks that are very sharp, sweet or too cold can make nausea or sickness worse.

- If you are feeling sick when you wake up, make sure you take your time getting out of bed. If you can, have something to eat prior to doing so e.g. a dry biscuit, toast.

- Eat smaller meals, more regularly. Foods that are high in carbohydrate can help e.g. pasta, bread, crackers. Pregnant women often find savoury foods are tolerated well than spicy or sweet ones. NB: Don't stop eating! If you find the nausea and vomiting prevents you eating, you must consult your healthcare professional.

- Avoid smells or foods that make you feel sick. Some women find they prefer eating cold meals to hot ones, as they don't give off as much aroma. Ask someone else to do the cooking. If this is not an option, try to cook bland foods, like pasta, that don't give off too much of a smell and are easy to prepare.

- Sometimes the more you think about nausea the worse it can be, so try to find something distracting to do. Adjusting the clothing you wear can also help. Trade in your tight jeans for ones with a comfortable elastic waistband

- You may find that ginger products help to counteract nausea, but they are not licensed in the UK. Make sure you buy them from a reputable source, like a pharmacy. You might find that ginger biscuits or ginger ale help.

13. HOW DO I KNOW WHAT TRIMESTER I AM IN?

Your first quarter is going to be months one through three. Otherwise known as week zero to week thirteen. The second trimester is week fourteen to week twenty-seven months four to seven. Month seven to nine is the third quarter. It is week twenty-eight to when you give birth.

14. HOW MUCH WEIGHT SHOULD I GAIN WHILE PREGNANT?

Healthy weight gain for a pregnant woman is twenty-five to thirty-five pounds.

Should you be overweight, your weight gain is supposed to be around fifteen to twenty-five pounds.

If you are underweight, then it is safe for you to gain twenty-eight to forty pounds.

If you have multiple births, you should only gain about thirty-five to forty-five pounds.

15. IS GAS AND INDIGESTION NORMAL WHILE PREGNANT?

Yes. With the changes in hormones, the efficiency of the

gastrointestinal system is lowered. The first sign is going to be nausea and morning sickness probably. As your pregnancy progresses, it can change into acid reflux and indigestion. It is entirely reasonable.

16. WHEN WILL MY MORNING SICKNESS END?

For most women morning sickness stops at twelve weeks. However, some women end up having morning sickness until the end of their pregnancy.

17. WHAT ARE ACTIVITIES I SHOULD AVOID WHILE I AM PREGNANT?

You do not want to change the cat box. Doing this task can end up leading to complications for newborns.

- Paint. The exposure to the toxic chemicals is not okay for you or baby.
- Get an X-Ray unless you have to.
- Use a sauna, hot tub or tanning booth.
- Go on rides such as Great American Scream Machine or Tower of Terror.

18. WHAT CAN I DO TO RELIEVE OR PREVENT HEARTBURN?

To prevent heartburn, you should try and avoid greasy and spicy foods as well as drinks that contain a lot of caffeine. You can also try and eat smaller meals while avoiding having to bend or lay down right after you have eaten.

19. WHAT CAN I DO TO RELIEVE OR PREVENT LEG CRAMPS?

Make sure that you exercise regularly and are getting plenty of fluids in your system. It is also important that you do not sit in one position for an extended period. Massage your legs to keep blood flowing and apply heat when you need to relieve a cramp.

20. WHAT CAN I DO TO REDUCE OR PREVENT HAEMORRHOIDS?

Drink plenty of fluids and make sure that you have plenty of fibre in your diet. Exercising regularly and avoiding standing or sitting for extended periods of time. You can also try and take sitz baths while applying cold compresses to the affected area.

21. WHAT ARE SOME OF THE COMPLICATIONS THAT I CAN EXPERIENCE WHILE PREGNANT?

(a) Before Pregnancy:

As you are trying to get pregnant, you need to make sure you talk to your health care provider about any health issues you are currently going through or have experienced to make sure they do not cause any complications later in your pregnancy.

If the issue is current, then it may require you to change how you and your doctor are treating that problem due to the medication possibly causing a problem later on.

Also, it is important that you identify any issues that you had in previous pregnancies to try and get them addressed and possibly avoid them with this pregnancy.

(b) During Pregnancy:

 (c) Pregnancy Complications:

Urinary Tract Infection (UTI): this is a bacterial infection that occurs in your urinary tract. Signs that you have a UTI are:

- Nausea or back pain

- Fever, tiredness, shakiness

- Pressure in your lower stomach

- Urine that smells bad or looks cloudy or reddish

- An urge to use the bathroom often

- Pain or a burning sensation when you go to the bathroom.

Should you believe that you have a UTI, it is important that you talk to your doctor about being tested. If you test positive, then your doctor will be able to give you a treatment of antibiotics so that you can kill the infections to make it better in a day or two.

(d) Anemia:

It is when there is a lower number of red blood cells than what you should have in your body. When you are being treated for the underlying cause of anaemia, then you will be able to restore the number of healthy red blood cells. There is a possibility that you will feel tired as well as weak should you have anaemia. It can be treated by taking folic acid and even iron supplements.

(e) Mental Health Conditions:

You may even experience depression while you are pregnant. If your depression persists throughout your entire pregnancy, you may want to consider talking to a therapist to help you get your depression treated. Depression can end up causing you to have trouble taking care of your baby after they are born.

A few other complications that you may come across are obesity and weight gain, infections, high blood pressure, hyperemesis gravidarum (morning sickness/nausea), or GDM (Gestational Diabetes Mellitus).

22. IS THE BLEEDING CAUSE FOR ALARM WHILE I AM PREGNANT?

Yes! Bleeding can mean that complications are occurring in your pregnancy and you need to be seen immediately.

Anything from zero to twenty weeks means that you could be

having a miscarriage.

Anything between twenty to thirty-seven weeks means that you could be having preterm labour

And at any time it could mean that there are problems with your placenta such as it has separated from the inner wall of your uterus.

23. HOW BAD WILL MY PREGNANCY DIZZINESS GET?

It is a common symptom to feel dizzy while you are pregnant. During your early pregnancy, it means that you could have low blood sugar and need to eat something. You may feel dizzy up until you give birth due to your uterus putting pressure on the arteries in your legs. However, always try and eat something to make sure it is not just low blood sugar.

24. HOW WILL I KNOW IF I AM IN LABOUR?

You will know you are in labour when you begin to experience

- Muscular contractions that are happening at short intervals,

- Your water has broken,

- You are having cramps in your lower back that are not going away,

- You have a bloody mucus discharge.

25. HOW DO I KNOW WHEN I AM READY TO PUSH?

You will push when you are experiencing a contraction after you have fully dilated. Your nurse or doctor will keep track of how far dilated you are and will tell you when it is safe for you to push and when it is not. You will not push when you are not having a contraction because that will just cause your labour to be harder than necessary.

26. HOW DO I KNOW IF THE TIME IS RIGHT TO BECOME PREGNANT?

Having a baby is a big step. If you are properly prepared, then you will find you will be less stressed while trying to conceive and during pregnancy. As they say, 'forewarned is forearmed.' Before you try to conceive, it is best to schedule an appointment with your doctor. They can carry out a general health check, and it is a chance for you and your partner to ask questions you may have, about pregnancy and childbirth. If you are on any regular medication or have a chronic illness, this is the time to discuss the issue with your doctor, and they can arrange for you to see a consultant. Moreover, your doctor can provide you with information in regards to folic acid, antenatal vitamins, and other steps to prepare your body for conception.

I have a baby?

Every woman looks at pregnancy differently. Therefore there will be very individual reviews/reactions. Some women seem to breeze through pregnancy. Others can experience entirely negative feelings, and this can be quite reasonable. It is a big step to take, and there is a lot to consider. Are you going to undergo antenatal screening? If you do and you receive unwelcome results, how are you going to react/what is your next step?

27. WHAT TO DO IF NAUSEA AND VOMITING BECOME SEVERE?

If your nausea and vomiting becomes severe and does not respond to the remedies above, you might find your GP prescribes a short course of anti-sickness (antiemetic) medication. Some antihistamines (for allergies) can also help control sickness. Do not take anything unless it has been prescribed primarily for you!

28. WHAT SUPPLEMENTS SHOULD I TAKE BEFORE AND DURING PREGNANCY?

Folic Acid is a must as soon as you plan on becoming pregnant. You need to take 400 micrograms every day, while you are trying to conceive and up until you are 12 weeks. Why? Folic Acid can help to reduce neural tube defects, such as Spina Bifida. Obviously check with your midwife or doctor first, but you need to choose an antenatal vitamin that includes: Folic acid, vitamin D, calcium, vitamin C, thiamine, riboflavin, niacin, and vitamin B12.

29. WHEN WILL I START TO FEEL THE BABY MOVE?

Baby movement or 'quickening' is usually considered between weeks 16 to 25. In your first pregnancy, it might not be until closer to the 25 weeks. In a woman's second or subsequent pregnancy they may feel it at 13 weeks. Remember every woman is different but if you are at all concerned talk to your midwife or doctor.

30. WHAT MEDICATION CAN I TAKE WHILE I AM PREGNANT?

With any medication in pregnancy, whether supermarket or pharmacy bought you should discuss taking them with your doctor. Some herbal/alternative remedies are safe to take while pregnant to relieve things such as nausea. Some are not! So please check with your GP/midwife, before taking them. Also, make sure you adhere to the correct dose. Do not take an increased dose, thinking it will be more efficient!

31. WHY AM I EXPERIENCING HEADACHES, WHILE PREGNANT?

In early pregnancy, there is an increase in hormones and blood flow, and this may mean more frequent headaches. Other causes can be stress, low blood sugar, tiredness and dehydration. Later in pregnancy, they tend to be caused due to poor posture. Whatever the cause, before you take any medication to combat them, talk to your GP first.

32. WHY AM I GETTING LOWER BACK PAIN?

Your body produces a hormone (relaxin) that causes the ligaments in your pelvic area to relax. It may also cause ligaments in your spine to loosen, which can cause pain. Your spine supports the extra weight gained during pregnancy, and your growing uterus puts pressure on nerves and blood vessels in your back and pelvis. Your centre of gravity changes due to weight gain later in pregnancy, so you may start to modify the way you stand/move to compensate. Trying the following may help Regular exercise, to strengthen muscles and to improve your flexibility; improved posture (make sure you don't slouch). Changing the way, you sit, and sleep can also help to ease any back pain that you are feeling. If you sleep on your side, you may want to try placing a pillow between your knees.

33. ARE HEARTBURN AND INDIGESTION EVERYDAY WHILE PREGNANT?

Digestion is slowed down in pregnancy, due to progesterone making muscles smoother. The valve at the top of the oesophagus can also open or leak, which then lets stomach acid flow upwards. Also, as your uterus grows, it pushes on your stomach causing more pressure on the valve. To help avoid heartburn, try not to eat greasy or spicy foods, and drinks that contain a lot of caffeine. You can also try and eat smaller meals while avoiding bending or laying down right after you have eaten.

34. IS IT NORMAL TO HAVE OTHER DISCHARGE WHILE PREGNANT?

Yes, but it should be thin, white and usually odourless or mild smelling, and is caused by having extra blood flow going to your pelvis. If you find the discharge changes colour, smells looks unusual, or you experience pain, itching or soreness, contact your GP. It may mean you have thrush, and this is easily treated.

N.B: Do not use tampons while pregnant, as more germs may be introduced into your vagina.

35. HOW CAN I RELIEVE LEG CRAMPS?

No-one is exactly sure what causes leg cramps. But there are a few things you can do if you get them:

- Straighten your leg, then (gently) flex your toes and ankles towards your calf.

- Try standing on a cold surface, as this can sometimes stop a spasm

N.B: If the flexing or cold do not work, make sure you see you GP, immediately. In rare instances, the pain could be due to a blood clot. Do not massage, as this could make it worse.

36. CAN I PREVENT STRETCH MARKS

Stretch marks are caused, in later pregnancy due to changes in elastic tissue that is just below the skin's surface. Genetics can play a part in whether you get them or not. Although you may not be able to avoid them, you may be able to slow them down. No stretch mark cream is going to prevent them but massaging your skin, with oil or cream can help you to feel good, and it may even encourage new tissue growth.

CHAPTER 2: PREGNANCY AND NUTRITION QUESTIONS

37. WHAT IS THE FOOD I CANNOT EAT DURING PREGNANCY?

It is suggested that you need to stay away from:

- Fish that contains a lot of mercury. Having large amounts of mercury in your system can end up damaging a developing brain.

- You should also stay away from any unpasteurized soft cheeses such as brie, feta, gorgonzola, etc.

- Raw fish such as sushi.

- Cold ready to eat meals like hot dogs or lunch meat because of the listeria that the meat can contain.

- Unpasteurized milk (which is also a source of listeria).

- Alcohol because it can interfere with the development of your fetus and even lead to fetal alcohol syndrome.

- Uncooked or cured eggs and meats such as prosciutto, or runny eggs.

- Caffeine, however, it is okay when you take it in moderate amounts.

38. WHAT IS THE BEST NUTRITION FOR PREGNANT WOMEN?

Above all, you need to follow a healthy diet, and your body needs extra vitamins and minerals. Whatever anybody may tell you, you do not need to 'eat for two'. It is advised that you eat an extra 350 to 500 calories (1470 to 2090 kilojoules) during the 2nd and 3rd trimesters. If your diet is lacking, it may affect the baby's development.

Poor eating habits and gaining excess weight can put you at a higher risk of gestational diabetes, or birth complications. Things such as leafy greens, vegetables, fruits, whole grain bread and cereals are going to be the best option, while you are pregnant. You also need to consume food that contains protein and calcium, such as low-fat yoghurts, broccoli, eggs, and salmon. When it comes to meat, please refer to the section on what not to eat, but above all make sure the meat is cooked thoroughly!

39. DOES IT MATTER IF I MISS A DAY OF MY PREGNANCY VITAMINS?

Prenatal vitamins are important in helping to bridge the gap in any of the nutrients that you may be missing in your diet. However, if you happen to miss a day or two of your prenatal vitamins, you are not going to find that anything is going to happen to you or your baby. Some women never take prenatal vitamins when they are pregnant.

40. WHAT SHOULD I DO IF I BECOME CONSTIPATED DURING PREGNANCY?

Constipation is something that many pregnant women complain about. It is not too uncommon for women at some point in their pregnancy. With all the progesterone in your system, you are going to realise that your muscles are smoothed out and relaxed, and this also affects the digestive tract.

Due to all the progesterone, your food is going to pass through your digestive system slower. Not only that but taking iron supplements in high doses is going to cause you to have constipation.

To combat illness, you can:

(a) Drink plenty of water

Your urine should look bright. One glass of juice a day will help as well, most particularly prune juice to help regulate your digestive system. There have been reports that drinking some warm liquid after you get up will also contribute to keeping you from being constipated.

(b). Eat foods that are high in fibre

It should be things such as whole grain bread and cereals along with brown rice, beans, and fresh vegetables and fruits. You can also include a tablespoon or two of unprocessed wheat bran with your breakfast along with a glass of water to help you get things moving.

(c) Look at your prenatal vitamins

If they contain a high amount of iron, then ask your healthcare provider about switching to a different prenatal that does not have so much iron in it. The only reason that you need a lot of iron is that you are anaemic and are needing to increase your iron intake.

41. CAN I EAT A VEGETARIAN DIET WHILE PREGNANT?

Make sure you plan your meals and eat a variety of healthy,

nutritious vegetarian foods, then you should be able to continue. Make sure you consume all the necessary vitamins, minerals, protein and nutrients that you and your baby need. If in doubt, talk to your midwife or doctor.

42. DISPERSING YOUR MEALS DURING PREGNANCY

One of the best difficulties that many pregnant ladies confront is when to eat their dinners such that they keep up their optimal weight while eating for two.

Specialists suggest that as opposed to eating three substantial suppers for every day, one should attempt and eat around six little dinners rather, as this will lessen the odds of them putting on additional weight.

One motivation behind why pregnant ladies should prepare for putting on extra weight amid pregnancy incorporates the potential danger of creating diabetes or hypertension.

You likewise need to abstain from putting on an excessive amount of weight amid pregnancy since you will have more weight to lose after you are through with labour. Then again, you need to ensure that you eat enough nourishment with the goal that you put on simply enough weight to guarantee that your kid doesn't have a low fetal weight, or be conceived rashly.

Numerous positive advantages are identified with eating six little suppers consistently amid pregnancy. For instance, the difficulties you may confront from morning infection, or the weight from the developing embryo, won't enable you to eat as much as you may need to at any rate.

There is no better approach to stay aware of your suggested calorie admission than eating various little suppers in light of the trouble you will discover in eating a large dinner. You will likewise have the capacity to all the more effortlessly maintain a strategic distance from the compulsion to gorge, because of those raging hormones that can without much of a stretch increment your yearning.

Pregnant ladies will, usually, encounter instances of low glucose due to the way that the body forms it. Occurrences of low glucose in the body are ordinarily described by manifestations, for example, wooziness, shaking and discombobulation. In any case, you can go without much of a stretch balance out your glucose levels by guaranteeing that the six little dinners are equitably dispersed for the day while ensuring that they are preferably pressed with supplements that are solid.

Whenever possible, you may likewise need to expand the measures of low-fat proteins like poultry, grains, entire wheat bread, natural products, vegetables and skimmed drain.

43. SUSTENANCE'S YOU SHOULD AVOID AT ALL COSTS

Numerous ladies understand the significance of keeping up an all around adjusted eating routine amid pregnancy. You have to guarantee that you are getting all the basic vitamins, minerals and supplements, particularly for your creating child.

On the flip side, there are likewise nourishments that might be normal however perhaps ought to be best abstained from amid pregnancy. Some of these sustenances include:

• Raw meats: This will incorporate any undercooked hamburger, poultry or uncooked fish since they increment the odds of disease from salmonella, toxoplasmosis and also coliform microscopic organisms.

• Fish with large amounts of mercury: Try to control far from an angle that contains elevated amounts of mercury. There have been examples where youngsters conceived of ladies who expended large sums of mercury amid pregnancy are either mind harmed, or have developmental issues. You will consequently need to maintain a strategic distance from fish, for example, lord mackerel, swordfish, tilefish or shark and additionally sushi.

• Smoked fish: It is likewise realised that smoked fish that is refrigerated is additionally polluted with Listeria. You are well on the way to discover these nourishments in the shop area of numerous sustenance stores.

• Raw shellfish: Seafood that can cause sickness, for example, molluscs, clams, mussels and undercooked shellfish.

• Fresh eggs: You should maintain a strategic distance from every uncooked egg or sustenance's that contain them since they will doubtlessly be presented to salmonella. It will incorporate things, for example, hand crafted dessert, mayonnaise, custards or different sauces that are probably going to contain raw eggs.

• Soft cheeses: There is a probability that some foreign made fine cheeses are rearing reason for Listeria. You should check to guarantee that the cheddar you purchase is produced using sanitised drain.

• Unpasteurized drain: It is conceivable that any untreated waste you take may contain hazardous microscopic organisms that can prompt dangerous diseases.

• Caffeine: While right levels of caffeine ought to be alright, there are examiners that have connected a lot of caffeine taken by a pregnant lady to low birth weight, premature births, premature labours and additionally withdrawal side effects among newborn children.

• Alcohol: When it comes to liquor, not a single drop ought to be taken amid pregnancy, and like this you ought to stay away from it totally amid pregnancy. Alcohol is known to meddle with the advancement of the embryo in more routes than one. At times, it has been known to prompt fetal alcohol disorder and also various formative issue.

• Unwashed raw vegetables: While vegetables are among the most beneficial sustenance's you can consider eating, it is constantly essential to ensure that they are all around cooked. Crude vegetables might be sullied with toxoplasmosis, which is in some cases found in the dirt where the plants are developed.

44. VEGETARIANISM AND PREGNANCY

The most vital thing you should ensure you do amid your pregnancy is to eat a healthy eating routine. Ladies who eat solid will generally bring forth a sound infant.

While there is no genuine issue with vegan diets amid pregnancy, women who take after this eating routine must ensure that they get each supplement that is required amid pregnancy. Despite the fact that this can be a testing exercise, in truth, it should be possible.

A pregnant lady must see to it that she gets an adequate measure of protein, calcium, press, vitamin B12 and vitamin D. These are a portion of the supplements that can be a test, particularly for those ladies who are absolutely vegans. Amid your pregnancy, it is basic that you increment your protein allow by 25 grams day by day.

Lacto – Ovo veggie lovers, the individuals who eat eggs and drain as the primary creature items they expand can think that it's less demanding to expand the protein allow by having some drain, some additional cuts of cheddar or maybe an extra number of eggs.

Vegetarians then again, who rely upon plant sustenance's alone, should purposely build their protein allow to keep a reliable pregnancy.

Ladies likewise require a lot of iron in the midst of gestation and, much of the time, your specialist will prescribe some iron supplements.

The other thing that vegans must be watchful about is their utilisation of calcium, vitamin B12, and also vitamin D. It is anything but difficult to get your calcium from nourishments, for example, cheddar, yoghurt and drains or other option sources, for example, squeezed orange and strengthened breakfast oats. Extraordinary compared to other wellsprings of vitamin D is drinking reinforced drain while vitamin B12 can without much of a stretch be found in sustained oats.

With regards to vegetarians, extraordinary care must be taken because while you can get vitamin B12 from various ocean vegetables, tempeh or green growth, the volumes are ordinarily insignificant.

45. EATING SUSHI OR RAW FISH IS UNSAFE.

Eating sushi could be unsafe or possibly not. This relies on the kind of fish and the measure of fish utilised as a part of making the sushi. It resembles this; We know we need to attempt and abstain from having hazardous levels of mercury in our framework and hints of Mercury are found in general angle. Cooking does not expel the mercury, so it's best to eat a worthy add up to make sure that you will be protected.

On the off chance that you adore your raw fish sushi, it is

critical to attempt and evade huge fish, the bigger the fish, the more mercury there. These incorporate Shark, Swordfish, Marlin or Deep Sea Perch.

That is not by any means the only stresses with eating sushi. If you adore sushi with raw fish, there is the risk of contracting Hepatitis A, getting worms or parasites, or outright queasiness from getting raw fish that hasn't been put away legitimately.

So in case you're pregnant, it's likely better to evade the sushi with raw fish, and it is probably best to stay with those rolls containing cooked fish. Or, on the other hand, attempt Sushi that is principle fixings may be vegetables or even egg.

Ensure you arrange from a legitimate eatery that is utilising basic stockpiling and cooking strategies and total the sum that you eat.

46. AFTER YOU EAT, USE THE BATHROOM.

Your body knows when you need to get rid of the waste in it; so listen to it. Do not put off going to the bathroom once you feel the need to. Doing this can cause problems later on.

If all else fails, talk to your doctor about prescribing you something that can help or about adding an over the counter fibre supplement or even stool softener to your daily routine.

The only time that you should begin to worry about your constipation is if there are other symptoms with it such as, abdominal pain, you are passing mucus or blood, or you are having constipation and then diarrhoea alternating. At this point, you need to get in contact with your doctor or other health care provider as it may be a different issue that is causing this.

While you are going to the bathroom, try not to strain. If you strain, you can end up causing haemorrhoids or even cause them to worsen if you already have them. It is due by the swelling of the veins in your rectal area.

Hemorrhoids are painful and uncomfortable but will end up going away when you give birth to your baby. If you find that the pain is too severe or you have to bleed from your rental, you need to call your health care provider to see if there is a more serious issue going on.

CHAPTER 3: EXERCISE AND PREGNANCY QUESTIONS

47. WHAT EXERCISES CAN I DO WHILE I AM PREGNANT?

While you are pregnant, you can do activities such as swimming, walking, a stationary bike, low impact aerobics, a step machine, and even an elliptical machine. You can also do things such as tennis, racquetball, and jogging.

However, you need to be careful and talk to your health care provider if you are unsure if you should be doing the activity.

Exercise regularly

Doing light exercises such as swimming, yoga, riding a stationary bike, or even walking can help you to ease the pain of constipation and leave you not only feeling better but feeling healthier.

48. WHAT ARE MY EXERCISE LIMITATIONS WHILE I AM PREGNANT?

However, you are going to want to avoid things that are going to give you a higher risk of falling or any abdominal injury.

Along with those, you are going to want to avoid any high altitude sports.

49. NOURISHMENT AND EXERCISE

Diet will affect the well-being of your whole body, and accordingly, you require a legitimate eating regimen to support your odds at origination and a peaceful pregnancy.

It is constantly fitting that you take nutritious sustenances, mainly focusing on entire essential nourishments that must incorporate grains, nuts, fresh foods grown from the ground.

Most ladies have profited by changing to natural sustenances as a method for decreasing their potential admission of pesticides and other hurtful poisonous substances that are found in many prepared nourishments.

Through the assistance of your specialist you have to work towards your optimal body weight since being stout, or even underweight, can unfavourably influence pregnancy.

While overweight pregnant ladies open themselves to ailments, for example, diabetes and hypertension, the individuals who are underweight convey the danger of bringing forth low birth weight kids. Since it's past the point where it is possible to begin weight reduction or weight pick up diets after you imagine, a weighted design ought to be considered path before you start endeavouring considering.

As a pregnant lady or one who is endeavouring to end up noticeably pregnant, you have to get into some wellbeing exercise administration to keep your body as alive and well. Great use advances the well-being of the whole body, including expanding flow and lessening stress, both of which are useful for origination.

With a decent exercise design, you will likewise figure out how to shed off any overabundance calories, and also getting some solid rest, which will enable the body self to repair.

It is critical that you do your activity with some restraint because on the off chance that it is done unreasonably it can intrude on the body's hormonal adjust to such an extent that it disturbs your menstrual cycle and additionally ovulation.

You may profit a considerable measure by conversing with your specialist about the measure of activity you ought to do as such that it doesn't meddle with your menstrual cycle.

Over the top exercise can diminish the condition of ripeness. It can upset the healthy stream of hormones and meddle with ovulation and menstrual cycles, and subsequently influence fruitfulness.

That is the reason a few ladies who run more than 20 miles seven days have rare or truant menstrual cycles.

If your activity routine meddles with a typical month to month menstrual cycle, you'll need to diminish your exercise to get your body controlled before you can consider.

Converse with your specialist about how to best re-establish a sound hormonal adjust.

CHAPTER 4: LIFESTYLE AND PREGNANCY QUESTIONS

50. CAN I HAVE SEX WHILE I AM PREGNANT?

Yes!

Reassure him that he is not going to hurt you or the baby. If he is still unsure about it, then talk to your doctor about ways that you can help calm his fears so you can get back to doing what you want to do.

51. WHAT IS FIRST-TRIMESTER SCREENING?

It is a test that is done early in your pregnancy to offer some information about the chromosomal risks for things such as Down syndrome. Testing is done by either a blood test or by an ultrasound exam.

52. WHAT DO I DO WITH MY FIRST-TRIMESTER SCREENING RESULTS?

Your results are going to tell you if your baby is at risk for Down syndrome. This test does not mean that your child will have Down syndrome, it only shows you danger of carrying a baby with this genetic condition.

53. DOES YOUR PARTNER ALSO WANT A BABY?

"I truly need to have a child yet he doesn't" is a typical circumstance that a few couples need to manage.

While you may think needing a child is a unique feeling for all men and ladies, the reality of the situation is that there are individuals who essentially don't. While it might give the idea that your accomplice is rude or childish, you can't just constrain him to have one.

Rather than endeavouring to job openings in his condom or discover another person to make you pregnant, attempt to determine why he is impervious to having a child.

You should recollect that you ought not to compel your accomplice to have a child with you. Because you need a child does not imply that every one of your wants must be satisfied instantly. You youngster will be in an ideal situation on the off chance that it comes when both of you concur that it is the correct thing to do or maybe the perfect time to have one.

One essential thing you should consider is that you can't drive your man to need everything that you do or if nothing else in the meantime. Numerous ladies need to control their accomplice's decisions particularly on the off chance that they are hitched. You may have all the great purposes behind requiring a child right now however if your accomplice is loath to the thought; you might need to hold it until the point when you have a shared understanding.

A decent relationship is one where you acknowledge your accomplices wants recently like you would need him to answer yours. There are circumstances where your man may offer into your undue weight for requiring a youngster yet in truth this won't twist drill too well for your kid and also your relationship. Since your companion is relied upon to love, look after and furthermore bolster the youngster you truly need to have, you need to keep away from any circumstance where your tyke will feel undesirable as it grows up.

54. THE EFFECT OF PREGNANCY ON LIFESTYLE AND CAREER

While pregnancy can be an upbeat time for most ladies, it is additionally joined by various entanglements that will by and large influence your life in more routes than one.

One of the greatest things you will yield is the opportunity that you delighted in before origination. You should remember that you will never again have the capacity to appreciate the opportunity of being joyful and single since you will have an infant to deal with for a long time to come.

Getting pregnant implies that, not at all like when you were single, there will be confinements concerning your drinking, smoking (on the off chance that you do) and also dietary propensities. Amid those first long stretches of pregnancy, you may battle with the state of mind swings, sickness, push and furthermore intermittent shortcoming and so on. There will be numerous exercises you will most likely be unable to do, and also places, you will probably be unable to go to.

The minute you choose to get pregnant will mean you are entering an entirely new period of your way of life that you may have never envisioned. This new way of life will include various bargains you should make concerning your exercises all through, and even after, the kid arrives.

There might be limitations in regards to your voyaging, going to your wellness club or even the measure of work you will have the capacity to do as the pregnancy advances.

You will likewise need to recall that pregnancy could incredibly influence your association with your accomplice in some critical ways. Your life might be less sentimental than it was initially and sometimes you may even face limitations concerning your sexual contact amid pregnancy. Numerous ladies understand that pregnancy makes a passionate separation with their life partner, which was not foreseen.

Your profession is likewise going to get hammered in some basic courses as a result of your pregnancy. You may get frustrated when your specialist recommends an aggregate bed rest at what you may consider a vital phase of your vacation. While this may not be the standard, there are a couple of ladies who encounter complexities amid pregnancy such that they are compelled to give up their vacation incidentally.

There are a sizeable number of ladies who get discouraged when they understand that they need to hold their vocation for a timeframe to enable them to observe their pregnancy through to its decision securely.

In any case, many more ladies won't have any intricacies whatsoever.

55. IS IT ACCURATE TO SAY THAT YOU ARE EMOTIONALLY PREPARED FOR THE BABY?

Concluding that you will have a kid is maybe one of the life's most necessary decisions you will ever make.

It is on account of being a parent will change your life in more courses than you will ever envision. Most ladies ponder whether they have what it takes to start their adventure into parenthood.

Usually, many enthusiastic sentiments will spin somewhere inside you bringing an intricate blend of want, foresight and nervousness.

Since child rearing is full-time work, it is critical to contemplate around a couple of way of life and serious subject matters previously you choose to get pregnant. You and your mate should concur on a couple of critical issues to determine whether you are sincerely arranged to deal with a youngster.

It is exceptionally fundamental for future guardians to experience snapshots of uncertainty with many inquiries that will require answers. A portion of the queries you may need answers to keeping in mind the end goal to check whether you are candidly arranged to have a kid include:

• Whether you and your accomplice truly need a kid

• Whether you can bring up a tyke all alone if you are not in a perpetual relationship

• Whether you are set up for the path in which your pregnancy and tyke will influence your way of life, training and profession designs

• How you and your accomplice will manage any issues, for example, religious, racial or perhaps ethnic contrasts that could impact how your tyke is raised

• How you will manage issue of childcare

• Whether you are set up to bring up a youngster who is unwell or maybe one that requires extraordinary necessities

• If you are set up to relinquish your flexibility for the welfare of your youngster

• Whether you can envision yourself getting a charge out of child rearing

56. SETTING UP YOUR BODY FOR PREGNANCY

A standout amongst the most intriguing things about getting pregnant that many individuals underestimate is the need to plan for the expected pregnancy. Indeed, it is critical to understand the significance of setting up your body route before you start attempting to imagine.

Once your body is set up for pregnancy, you increment you odds of imagining from the word go.

Extraordinary compared to other approaches to get ready is to start by an eating regimen change to incorporate a plenitude of organic products, vegetables, entire grains and dairy items.

It is likewise critical to consider expanding your admission of lean proteins with a specific end goal to fabricate your stores, and however much as could be expected, go for natural nourishments, so you steer far from a significant number of the hazardous chemicals, pesticides and additives found in many handled sustenance's today.

Unless you get pregnant unintentionally, you should consider stopping the anti-conception medication technique you have been utilising to empower origination.

How soon you will feel could be halfway controlled by the sort of contraception you have been utilising. You ought to in this way not get restless on the off chance that you don't end up noticeably pregnant instantly you quit employing contraception:

• Birth control pills: If you have been employing conception prevention pills your body could start ovulating quickly or conceivably take a while before it at last starts.

• IUD: Women who have been on an Intra Uterine Device should have a specialist evacuate it, the outcome being that their bodies are prepared for origination very quickly.

• Barrier techniques: Women who utilise obstruction strategies, for example, spermicides, stomachs or condoms stay prolific whenever they don't use them. That these ladies should only to hurl aside whatever boundary they have been utilising, and they are prepared to take off running.

What you should recollect is that pregnancy can be contrasted with a marathon that takes a whole nine months.

You can improve the odds of having an inconvenience free

pregnancy by ensuring that your body, and particularly your regenerative framework, are fit as a fiddle before you even endeavour considering. That way, you will prime up your body, and your kid, for a decent begins in the marathon of life.

57. THE IMPORTANCE OF PRECONCEPTION SCREENING FOR INFECTIONS

Each lady who is anticipating getting to be plainly pregnant requirements to converse with her specialist about previously established inclination screening to check for any contaminations that could hinder her well-being and that of her infant.

It has turned into a major necessity since when a few sicknesses are dealt with and overseen early, the specialist dangers to the potential mother and the hatchling are lessened.

The motivation behind why this type of screening is imperative is that there are ladies who can convey a few sicknesses without demonstrating any indications.

The perfect time to lead the greater part of these blood tests is preceding getting to be plainly pregnant because, in situations where treatment or inoculations might be required, it is consistently protected to do them before one is pregnant. It is on account of there are immunisations that could show well-being dangers the embryo.

While there are standard blood tests that are ordinarily prescribed for every single pregnant lady, there are specific tests that will be performed on women who are in danger of specific infections.

A portion of the specified routine tests incorporates blood gathering and free response screening, rubella counter acting agent status, syphilis serology and midstream pee tests. Different tests will include ones for viral contaminations, for example, hepatitis B, hepatitis C, and also the Human Immunodeficiency Virus.

The other vital screening will be the cervical cytology test known as PAP spread.

58. UNENDING DISEASES AND HOW THEY CAN AFFECT YOUR PREGNANCY

Regarding the matter of real well-being amid pregnancy, various things should be mulled over, including a way of life, nourishment, physical wellness and also any probability of ceaseless maladies.

If you are endeavouring to get pregnant and you are living with infections, for example, diabetes, hypertension and asthma, among others, it would be a smart thought to illuminate your specialist previously.

You need to maintain a strategic distance from any dubious circumstances that these sicknesses could convey to your pregnancy or any potential damage to your healthy child. Your specialist should comprehend what drugs you are bringing together with their measurements, previously he or she would advise being able to you properly.

As a rule, the specialist will recommend various tests that will help her settle on an educated choice in regards to your mission for getting pregnant.

Your specialist will be in a position to enable you to deal with your pregnancy on the off chance that you have any constant maladies and furthermore stay away from any inconveniences. Ladies with uncontrolled diabetes will experience severe difficulties imagining, and now and again it is known to cause premature deliveries, or maybe notwithstanding passing some natural birth imperfections to the youngster.

While it remains a test to precisely know how pregnancy may impact asthma, near 25% of pregnant ladies with asthma find that their condition intensifies as of now.

Other interminable sicknesses that are known to bring confusions to pregnant ladies and their unborn children well-being incorporate hypertension, which is identified with instances of kidney issues.

Your heart gets an additional workload of around half amid pregnancy, and like this your specialist has to know whether you have a heart condition.

Make a point to converse with your specialist before getting to be noticeably pregnant on the off chance that you are experiencing any kidney ailment, urinary bladder difficulty, thyroid organ infection, iron deficiency, lupus or any malignancy.

59. Managing Genetic Disorders from Either of the Parents

Having an infant carries with it its particular offer of shocks, and particularly for the individuals who are doing it surprisingly.

Fortunately these days there is a large number of logical information out there that can help expel a lot of the mystery.

By embracing a proper eating regimen and going to pre-birth centres, you can make certain of having a healthy kid. Moreover, it is currently conceivable to comprehend what's in store through assumption screening.

Assumption genetic testing ends up plainly necessary, particularly in those situations where one of you is probably going to be inclined to specific conditions in light of their family line or even ethnic foundation. It is likewise fitting for you to visit a hereditary advisor assuming either or both of you expect that you could be conveying some genetic issue. You need to have genuine feelings of serenity by considering all your chances and alternatives because, as the familiar maxim goes, "better to be as careful as possible."

You might need to consider doing previously established inclination genetic screening on the off chance that you are:

• African-American: For sickle cell sickliness

• African, Mediterranean or Far East drop: For Thalassemia

European Jewish fall: Genetic blood issue particularly Tay-Sachs infection

• European Caucasian drop: For cystic fibrosis, although all couples ought.

• Women from families with history of hereditary issue: these incorporate issue, for example, haemophilia or robust dystrophy

While a few people may get restless at going for previously established inclination screening, it remains an ideal approach to evacuate any questions.

60. PRE-BIRTH VITAMINS AND SUPPLEMENTS

You more likely than not heard individuals say that the best time to deal with your child is enough before it arrives, or to be exact, even before you intend to wind up noticeably pregnant.

Fortunately, this is not a genuinely troublesome errand since you should simply pop some pre-birth vitamin or supplement and it's finished.

The advantage of this sort of program is that you will be loading the body with those supplements that are essential for origination and pregnancy.

The dominant part of these pre-birth vitamins contain folic corrosive, which is otherwise called folate, and an adequate measure of folic corrosive before origination has been demonstrated to decrease odds of a youngster being conceived with no imperfections, for example, spine bifida among others.

It is enough suggested that each lady who is of childbearing age should utilise 400mcg of folic corrosive every day regardless of whether they intend to get pregnant.

Women who originate from family lines with a past filled with deformities, for example, spine bifida need to take no less than 4mg of folic corrosive keeping in mind the end goal to diminish any odds.

Logical research demonstrates that when ladies take their day by day measurements of pregnancy related multivitamins, for example, vitamin B6 before they consider ordinarily endure fewer scenes or heaving and queasiness, otherwise called morning infection.

Other pre-birth supplements that contain minerals, for example, zinc are known to expand your fruitfulness levels.

61. CONVERSING WITH YOUR OBSTETRICIAN

Imagine a scenario where you Get Pregnant While Taking Contraceptives.

Anti-conception medication pills stay to be a standout amongst the most mainstream types of contraception with a huge number of ladies popping the pill around the world.

If these pills are taken by their guidelines, they give a 99% confirmation that you won't get pregnant.

Be that as it may, there are a few events where a lady will, in any case, consider while as yet taking anti-conception medication pills. The reasons why this may happen are fluctuated and may incorporate something a woman did or did not do or maybe the poll neglected to work for some reason.

A standout amongst the most widely recognised reasons why a conception prevention pill could ignore to work incorporates neglecting to take the pill on one or maybe more days. At times ladies are on such a bustling calendar, to the point that taking their pills will effectively slip their memory while they are still sexually dynamic.

The other reason this may happen is that a lady may change the time at which she takes the pill while it ought to be required at a similar investment every day.

While it might seem troublesome to need to take an anti-conception medication pill at about a same time every day, this is the main way that anti-conception medication pills will forestall pregnancy. The best thing you ought to do when you understand that you overlooked is to call your human services supplier and request their recommendation. Your social insurance vendor will have the capacity to instruct the best course concerning activity, contingent upon the specific pill you are taking.

There are those restless minutes when you have gone a long way from home and understand that you neglected to pack your pills. On the off chance that this happens, don't be enticed to take one given to you by a companion, since it may not work. The reality of the situation is that distinctive anti-conception medication pills have their remarkable details, and like this what has been recommended for another person may not work for you.

It is likewise conceivable that your conception prevention pill fizzled as a result of the impact of some other prescription you could be taking. There are specific drugs, for example, anti-infection agents, antifungal pharmaceuticals, and also hostile to seizure medicines that can entirely disable the power of conception prevention pills. It may likewise incorporate various natural items, and added vitamins and supplements.

It is in this manner vital to inform your specialist concerning any pharmaceutical you are taking to stay away from any potential outcomes of their checking.

Likewise, you have to understand that the contraception pill you swallow will take near 30 minutes before it is retained into the circulatory system. That inherently implies that you could get pregnant if your regurgitation before it has been maintained.

It is additionally a probability when you are experiencing extreme looseness of the bowels. On the off chance that you addressed your specialist about this he could really exhortation whether it is protected to take another pill.

Be that as it may, there is no compelling reason to stress over the security of your infant if you consider while still on a contraception pill. There is little confirmation that the hormones display in the contraceptive medicines can make any mischief the embryo.

Should this happen, you have to quit taking the pill and converse with your social insurance supplier.

62. IS YOUR AGE APPROPRIATE FOR PREGNANCY?

While getting to be plainly pregnant and bringing forth a tyke is viewed as a diagnostic procedure, there are times when specialists will be worried that yours is a high-chance pregnancy because of your age.

It is typical for ladies who are past the age of 30 to begin encountering a decrease in their ripeness level.

Women who are past the age of 35 are inclined to more dangers related with pregnancy and labour, thus the term high hazard pregnancy.

The issue of age related fruitfulness decay might be because of various things; hormonal changes are bringing about an adjustment in ovulation, a lessening of the quality and number of eggs, a decrease in the recurrence of sexual contact or maybe the nearness of other gynaecological conditions.

While it is moderately protected to wind up noticeably pregnant after 35 these days, there are various ripeness and pregnancy related difficulties that lady after 35 confront. It is hence vital for a girl who gets pregnant after the age of 35 to comprehend her hazard level and take enough prudent steps to lessen the potential dangers for the mother and the youngster.

There are various dangers related with endeavouring to imagine past 35 years old as the likelihood of birth abandons increment with a lady's age. For instance, while just 1 in each 1400 infants destined to women in their 20's is probably going to build up Down's Syndrome, the proportion lessens to 1 in each 100 kids for moms who are over the age of 35.

Ladies who are over 35 years likewise convey a higher danger of premature labour; while the proportion for women in their 20s is between 12% to 15%, this apportions increments to near 25% for females over the age of 40. The improved number of instances of irregularities could be identified with chromosomes, which is well on the way to happen in more established ladies.

There are a few different intricacies that will make pregnancy after 35 a high-chance pregnancy, for example, frequencies of endless well-being inconveniences, for example, hypertension and diabetes.

It is likewise more probable for ladies beyond 35 years old to encounter stillbirths, low birth weight babies, and more prominent odds of having your first kid by Cesarean Section.

Generally speaking of the thumb, high well-being before you

end up noticeably pregnant will incredibly lessen the chances of you having any real entanglements.

63. PICKING A GOOD OBSTETRICIAN AND MIDWIFE NURSE

As your pregnancy advances, sooner or later you should begin considering, and deciding, concerning where your child will be conveyed.

There are various decisions accessible to you as your pregnancy advances to term, and having a decent well-being expert will enable you to choose which decisions with bunches of certainty. One unusual choice will be whether to go for an obstetrician or a birthing specialist nurture.

The greater part of ladies has a tendency to pick obstetricians to enable them with their birthing to understanding. Obstetricians are exceptionally qualified experts who can without much of a stretch manage any conditions identified with the birthing knowledge from pregnancy the distance to the conveyance. It is additionally the favoured proficient ought to yours be a high-hazard pregnancy. As a rule, you will discover that your gynaecologist is likewise an obstetrician accordingly making things much less demanding for you.

A birthing specialist nurture then again will in all likelihood relate with you as a man, and not really as a patient. They can instruct you altogether about the regular birthing procedure, and they are additionally very prepared to manage any birth that is not confused. Much of the time they will allude your case on the off chance that they think there will be any confusions.

Extraordinary compared to other approaches to pick an obstetrician or maternity specialist nurture is through informal. You might need to address companions and relatives who might be more than willing to suggest experts they know. Be that as it may, you might need to ask your planned expert the accompanying inquiries too:

• When they think C-segments could be vital

• Under what conditions they perform episiotomies

• What healing facilities he or she conveys at

• How advantageous their office or healing facility is for conveyances

• Whether they convey alone or act as a significant aspect of a gathering

• Whether they are secured by your protection design

How Flexible is Your Health Care Provider?

Something that will help with your pregnancy and birthing knowledge has an obstetrician that you can be extremely open with.

Numerous years prior, picking an obstetrician was no major ordeal because there were truly no alternatives. By and large, all that a lady was keen on was getting a specialist who will help her and simply that.

Back then, they didn't have any pleasant birthing places, or even unique birthing methodology, for example, birthing

The experience of dealing with a certified midwife nurse is more likely to result in natural childbirth. While certified midwife nurses are known to be flexible, it is still possible to find an obstetrician with whom you could have a 'friendly' as opposed to a 'patient' type of relationship.

You may also want to find out if the health care practitioner you are dealing with will be able to deliver your baby at the hospital of your choice. You may have good reasons for choosing a particular hospital, maybe because of the amenities they provide for example.

Remember that you will be in that hospital for a few days and as a result, you need to be in an environment, you will love being in. You will most likely have toured the hospital in advance and looked at their rooms, as well as noted what rules they have so that you are sure they will make your birthing experience an unforgettable one.

64. ARE YOU A CANDIDATE FOR A C-SECTION?

While there are many women today choosing to have C-sections for various personal reasons, such as fear of pain or trying to avoid disrupting their programs, it is also true that much more have to undergo C-sections as a matter of necessity.

There are even many fourth time mothers who react to having to undergo C-sections with disappointment and shock because it was not part of their plans.

As a pregnant woman, you need to be aware of situations that could make a C-section necessary. You are most likely to undergo a C-section if you find yourself in any of the following categories:

☐ Overweight: Obese women have greater chances of suffering C-sections. It is because they are most likely to spend more hours during the first stages of labour than those who are of average weight. Having excess weight also increases chances that you could develop high blood pressure or diabetes during pregnancy, which will inadvertently increase the likelihood that you will undergo a C-section.

☐ Older than 40: The majority of women who are over the age of 40 when having their first child are candidates for C-section. Age brings with it a good share of pregnancy related complications, and some women beyond the age of 35 may have undertaken some form of fertility treatment, which will also increase the chances of a high-risk pregnancy.

☐ Multiple births: Having multiple births can also increase the likelihood that you will undergo a C-section, even though most of the time it will depend on the way the babies are lying in the womb.

☐ You have developed pre eclampsia: Close to 5% of pregnant women will develop preeclampsia, the symptoms of which are high blood pressure and a high level of protein in the urine. When there is a high standard of protein in the urine, it can cause a situation where there is a reduced flow of blood, which can harm the baby.

☐ Your child is in breech position: A baby is in a breech position when it has not yet turned correctly and is positioned feet or buttocks first. Your doctor will try to turn the baby, but if there is a likelihood of complication, C-section remains the way to go.

☐ You have had a previous C-section: Most women who have undergone C-section in previous births are generally encouraged to undergo the same to avoid chances of uterine rupture.

Any woman who has any of the above conditions is most likely going to be a candidate for C-section, and as such, you may need to plan appropriately. The good news is that C-sections can be safe so long as you get competent health care and support.

65. IS IT SAFE TO FLY WHILE PREGNANT?

If you are only having one baby, and your pregnancy has been a healthy one, then you can usually fly up until you're 36 weeks pregnant. Some airlines are reluctant to carry women after 28 weeks, due to the risk they may go into premature labour, so check with the individual airline. If you have a high-risk pregnancy, your doctor may advise you not to fly throughout your pregnancy.

It is perilous to fly amid the first trimester of pregnancy.

Except specific exemptions that I will say later, it is sheltered to fly amid your first trimester.

The likelihood of morning affliction, particularly if you as of now experience the ill effects of it could show up amid the flight since it happens whether you happen to be flying or not. Make certain to request a regurgitation sack if there isn't one as of now at your seat. Bringing moist toilettes from home to be ready is a smart thought.

The individual cases to flying in the first trimester would be anybody having any entanglements related to their pregnancy or who are thought to be 'high hazard'. It incorporates ladies with ineffectively controlled diabetes, sickle cell malady, placental variations from the norm, hypertension or those in danger of previous work. The absence of course can be an issue whether a man is pregnant or not. Move around the lodge of your plane to get a little exercise. It will help keep a course issue. Extend your legs under the seat in front of you and sporadically and pivot your lower legs. Folding your legs will add to the absence of flow, so endeavour to stay away from it.

Seats in planes appear to be getting littler which may make it awkward to move around. Inquire as to whether they have roomier seats and potentially pick one of those. It will add to your solace factor.

On account of metal indicators, they don't radiate x-beams, so there is no damage to you or your child's well-being.

It doesn't hurt to get some information about issues like this one. Be that as it may, for the most part, first trimester women can take off. Proceed, have a ball, it will benefit you.

66. COCOA BUTTER/MOISTURIZER WILL AVOID EXTENDING MARKS.

For a considerable length of time, we have all been advised amid pregnancy to slather ourselves with cocoa margarine to keep away those unattractive stretch marks.

Specialists have discovered that perhaps while facilitating our brains and alleviating our skin might be pleasant, there is no proof that cocoa margarine keeps extending checks away. An investigation was distributed in 2008 by a group of dermatologist and obstetricians that educated members to apply cocoa spread every day and another gathering to utilise a fake treatment. After numerous months, the scientists found no distinction in the seriousness of the extend checks by any means.

An agreeable woman in the primary need line was remarking on how cocoa margarine didn't shield her from getting marks, including that her young child had once raised the back of her shirt out in the open and said so anyone might hear, "Mother, how could you get those tiger stripes?"

Chuckling, she stated, "I don't care for having them. However I know with time they will likely blur."

In the off chance that you have outrageous extend marks, or can't stand seeing them, attempt vitamin E or a cream containing Alpha tocopherol. These have been observed to be more viable, however not by in particular.

Also, if cost is no issue, ask about radio frequency medications or surgery. Maybe we should only leave those separate checks be and see them as grand tiger stripes until the point when they blur away.

67. HAIR COLOURS ARE RISKY FOR THE CHILD.

Here's an inquiry that many ladies need to know the response to, because such a large number of us have a 4 to 6-week official date with the case of excellence. We may feel sick amid our initial three months of pregnancy yet that doesn't prevent the vast majority of us from needing to look impressive, particularly when it's our hair. It is what the American College of Obstetricians and Gynecologist need to state: Hair colours are most likely safe to use amid pregnancy since so little colour is retained through the skin.

In any case, it is as yet imperative to be mindful. Subsequently numerous therapeutic services suppliers suggest that pregnant ladies not utilise permanent hair colours amid the initial three months. While the retention through the skin is insignificant, the worry is that breathing the exhaust amid the procedure could be unsafe to the creating embryo. Perpetual hair colours contain smelling salts which have a solid concoction rage. It is best to dodge hair colours that contain alkali. Semi-changeless colours or featuring is viewed as more secure. With features, the thwart utilised keeps the colour from sitting on your head and won't be consumed. Henna and vegetable colours are additionally viewed as protected to utilise.

Here are a few recommendations:

Consider sitting tight until the point that the second trimester for hair colour, fading, permanents or fixing.

Do a fixed test for unfavourably susceptible responses previously finishing the procedure Open windows, work with a fan blowing or shaking your hair on your yard for good ventilation.

Make sure and set a clock and evacuate chemicals as the directions recommend. Flush your scalp thoroughly with water after treatment.

Continuously wear gloves and deliberately take after the headings on the item bundle.

What's more, as usual, ask your specialist or birthing assistant if you have any inquiries.

Lifting your arms over your head will make the umbilical line wrap around the infant's neck.

This old myth has been around for quite a while, yet doesn't have a leg (or an arm) to remain on. What could make the rope circumvent the child's neck? The arm is not associated with the string, nor does any weapon development influence the child inside the protected, fluid condition they are staying in.

Infants are regularly conceived with the rope around their neck, and today it is a fundamental thing for the specialist to unwrap it delicately. This not the slightest bit has anything to do with how you've moved or dozed or anything that you have done. On the off chance that it is okay to specialists for pregnant women to take Yoga, with every one of the positions that are required, one ought not to be worried about how she moves or does.

Some extraordinary activities and extend positions (through Yoga or Pilates) runs a danger of influencing the child, so ensure that you and your think supplier convey about any activities you need to do while pregnant. Be that as it may, lifting your arms over your head is not one of those.

So don't stress. If you have to achieve the plates that are far up there on the best retire, proceed, it won't make any mischief.

68. SHOWERS ARE PERILOUS FOR PREGNANT LADIES.

This likely began because while one is pregnant she might be somewhat less beyond any doubt on her feet, in light of various weight appropriation and adjusted focal point of gravity, and you could fall. It's imperative to be additional watchful while getting in the tub, and in the last trimester have somebody close by to help you.

Likewise having the water excessively hot could cause you, making it impossible to feel unsteady, which could add to the peril of falling.

It is what you have to know:

Ensure the water is lukewarm, so you don't overheat. You can sweat to chill, yet you're creating infant can't, so if the water is excessively hot for you, making it impossible to venture in ordinarily, it's most likely overly hot. (The general accord among guardians is to keep it underneath 100° F.) If you are experiencing squeamishness, abstain from utilising perfumed cleansers or creams. It may exacerbate queasiness. What's more, it's most likely best to stay with items that are free of colours, scents, and massive amounts of added substances since pregnant ladies are more inclined to urinary tract diseases and vaginal disturbance.

What's more, despite the fact that if you might be feeling muscle spasms and by and large achiness, ask your specialist or maternity specialist first before you utilise Epsom salts or some other shower added substance for torment.

69. ESPRESSO WILL CAUSE SKIN PIGMENTATIONS OR IS AWFUL FOR THE CHILD.

It is one myth that isn't heard all that regularly any longer, maybe because it is excessively abnormal, making it impossible to accept. Be that as it may, despite everything it comes up from time to time: if a lady drinks espresso while pregnant, it will make the infant have a skin pigmentation.

Approve, we should get the realities about skin pigmentations. As a matter of first importance, there are a few distinct sorts of skin pigmentations. Some are red, pink, or purple which are caused by abnormal platelets under the skin. Others are darker, created by the grouping of pigmented cells.

Frequently, skin colourations are minor injuries of veins caused by the weight that is put on the infant amid birth. Port wine recolour skin pigmentations' reasons differ, and there is a wrangle over mainly what causes them. Be that as it may, one thing is sure: there is no relationship amongst espresso and pigmentations.

It is valid, in any case, that when pregnant, ladies ought to most likely break point their admission of espresso to two glasses every day in light of the caffeine content. As new research rises, experts are finding that caffeine in extraordinary sums while pregnant have been connected with brought down birth weight and other, scarier issues. Converse with your parental figure if you have any worries about your caffeine admission.

Along these lines, on the off chance that you appreciate espresso, drinking it wouldn't stamp your child in any capacity. What's more, there is dependably decaf.

CHAPTER 5: YOGA AND PREGNANCY QUESTIONS

70. WHAT ARE THE BENEFITS OF YOGA DURING PREGNANCY?

Yoga amid pregnancy is typically alluded to among Yoga buffs as pre-birth Yoga. Any expecting mother who is endeavouring to get pregnant or at some phase over the span of pregnancy needs to do anything she can to influence this important time to go well. Your anxiety for the soundness of your unborn youngster is normal. Furthermore, it's okay to be worried about the massive physical and enthusiastic changes that happen to your body when you bring another life into this world. It is an excellent affair for any lady however it is likewise one that can cause stress and some inconvenience end route.

If you as of now are dynamic in the utilisation of Yoga before getting pregnant, you know the benefit of it. Your worries at that point are whether it is savvy to keep on participating in Yoga earlier and amid the different phases of pregnancy. Fortunately, the well-being and the estimation of pre-birth Yoga have been examined commonly, and the outcomes are very positive. The advantages of Yoga amid pregnancy have been archived, and the findings demonstrate that Yoga can be an enormous benefit to the unborn tyke and the mother all through your pregnancy term.

A 2005 investigation of more than 300 pregnant ladies found that the constructive outcomes of Yoga amid pregnancy on the unborn youngster were astounding and exceptionally active. Infants conceived of moms who rehearsed Yoga for only an hour a day had quantifiably higher birth weights. Intricacies amid pregnancy and work for such ladies and children were additionally discernibly lower. Specific issues like pregnancy-actuated hypertension and secluded intrauterine development impediment were limitless to a lesser degree a problem for infants of mothers who were understudies of Yoga.

The uplifting news proceeds when additional investigations investigated the impact of Yoga on the well-being of ladies earlier and amid their pregnancy. A different report in Thailand in 2008 found that ladies who rehearse Yoga routinely all through their pregnancy had a significantly more pleasant time amid work and their work time was shorter than females who had not been a piece of the Yoga encounter. Amid the nine months of pregnancy, an all-around composed Yoga program likewise assisted with the numerous physical challenges of pregnancy.

Ladies who were a piece of a pre-birth Yoga program experienced much-decreased frequencies of sciatica, swelling, spinal pain wrist torment, hip inconvenience, and even sickness.

What's more, since Yoga is likewise a mental and otherworldly teach, ladies who were consistent understudies of Yoga all through pregnancy felt less tension, rested better and had an overall more positive mental standpoint all through this necessary time in their lives and the lives of their children.

Regardless of the possibility that you were not an understudy of Yoga before beginning your pregnancy, that ought not to keep you down. If anything, the advantages of Yoga for you as an eager mother and for your pre-birth youngster are profound to the point that i

71. YOGA AND THE STAGES OF PREGNANCY

The advantages of Yoga amid pregnancy are clear. On the off chance that you have not been presented to Yoga, it could speak to anxiety. You are persuaded that you should figure out how to do Yoga for the benefit of your child and to influence your periods of pregnancy to go better. Now and then, in any case, it is anything but difficult to see the train of Yoga as unusual, extraordinary and confounding. Try not to let any misguided judgments you may have about Yoga shield you from getting the great advantages that Yoga can give to you amid your pregnancy.

One mistaken decision that ought to be shot down immediately is one that shields many individuals from investigating Yoga. Yoga is not a religion. You can appreciate the advantages of Yoga regardless of what your religious convictions are or on the off chance that you have no religious beliefs by any means. Doubtlessly Yoga became out of eastern religious controls, and it can turn into a piece of your private otherworldly life. The orders of Yoga are physical, mental and metaphysical. So as you learn great breathing strategies and how to utilise your body well amid your Yoga works out, that can turn out to be a piece of a single regimen of contemplation and reflection.

For a gigantic portion of the number of inhabitants in individuals who adore Yoga, the preparation can be useful isolate from any religious instructing. So you can simply ahead and take in more about how to move on a decent pre-birth Yoga program with no apprehensions. Yoga is additionally a preparing that is exceptionally adaptable. Try not to feel that you can't be a piece of a Yoga class if you are flabby or have never had accomplishment with work out. A decent Yoga coach will discover where you are and enable you to begin with the goal that you will start getting a charge out of the advantages of Yoga well before you wind up plainly gifted at the diverse Yoga works out.

Notwithstanding amid the way toward getting pregnant, Yoga can be a sound piece of your life. For couples who are experiencing issues or are chipping away at getting pregnant, it is anything but difficult to wind up plainly centred around each part of your physical life from what you eat to how well your clothing fits. On the off chance that a lady is dynamic in Yoga, at times there is a worry about whether the Yoga teach ought to be suspended as you attempt to begin your family.

As a general rule, having Yoga as a component of your week by week routine of activity is beneficial for you as you look for each way you can use to enable origination to occur. The active exercise of a standard Yoga class will empower blood stream and help your assimilation and end. It benefits your capacity to rest soundly and be completely casual. These things prompt a very much adjusted well-being picture for your body.

Most specialists will concur that the advantages of activity can resolve physical issues a mother to-be might be having and make the ordinary stride of getting pregnant less demanding to accomplish. Actually, on the off chance that you are looking to begin y your pregnancy and you need to achieve something useful for your body, starting another program of Yoga practice is an astounding stride the correct way.

It is dependably an intelligent thought to counsel with your specialist about how to fit Yoga into where you are in your pregnancy, and that starts with origination. Your specialist will know about any current issues you may have that ought to be thought about when beginning to take an interest in a Yoga class.

For a mother-to-be, fitting Yoga into your week by week timetable might be as much an issue of timing as it is about any worry about whether Yoga is a smart thought amid pregnancy. If you effectively dynamic in going to Yoga classes and getting a charge out of the advantages of Yoga every week, the inquiry might be if there will come a period when you should change or suspend your Yoga propensity in light of your pregnancy. Try not to be rushed in transforming anything even after you end up noticeably mindful that you are pregnant. For a certain something, your body is utilised to the activity, so you are insightful to proceed with that standard normal as your pregnancy gets in progress.

Furthermore, the advantage of having your body fit as a fiddle through the common interest in Yoga and the quality and capacity it gives will be used in each phase of pregnancy. As we specified before, be that as it may, there will come a period when it is insightful to change from your consistent Yoga class to a pre-birth Yoga class when you have a more unique need your Yoga program redid to fit your changing physical condition. Numerous ladies who are dynamic in a Yoga class ponder when the time is all in all correct to change to a class that is centred around expecting mothers.

There is not rigid control of when to change from your general Yoga class to a pre-birth Yoga setting. One incentive to beginning with a pre-birth Yoga class early is that you will meet other expecting mothers and you can experience the procedure together. One of the greatest preferences of being a piece of the Yoga people group is the social part of working out with other individuals who share your affection for Yoga. That is additionally something about changing from a standard Yoga class to pre-birth class that might be upsetting. You might be hesitant to leave your old Yoga class essentially because you like the general population you see there every week.

It merits putting in context. Your typical Yoga class is intended for general Yoga understudies so the activities can be as thorough as the teacher considers appropriate for his or her gathering. As your pregnancy moves along, you should move to a Yoga program that is intended for your physical condition. On account of that, your consistent class may never again be suitable for you.

As opposed to putting the duty on your typical Yoga educator to suit you so you can be with your companions, make that huge stride of exchanging classes. You will miss your friends from your old Yoga class and your former educator. However, they will all concur this is the best thing for you and your child. What's more, when you begin going to your pre-birth Yoga class, the certainty that you will be working with a Yoga teacher who is centred around pregnant mothers will more than beat the loss of association with your old class.

If you are new to the Yoga way of life, you are no uncertainty taking a gander at taking Yoga while you are pregnant for the many advantages we talked about before. You will be somewhat anxious however energised because this initial involvement with Yoga will open up a radically new world and it will make your pregnancy so significantly simpler and much more fun as you appreciate the encounters you have with your Yoga sessions.

For Yoga "novices", it bodes well to agree to accept a pre-birth Yoga class first thing, so you don't have progress to experience. If you only learned you are pregnant, there is no motivation to hold up. Truth be told, if you start to take in the different trains and activities of Yoga before your pregnancy is exceptionally far along, that will help you when those same events are altered to suit the adjustments in your body when you are conveying an unborn baby within you. Try not to be modest if you go to visit first pre-birth Yoga class and there are ladies there who are substantially further along in their pregnancies than you. Only make the most of your first experience of learning Yoga and let it turn into a propensity.

The odds are that it will end up being a long lasting tendency even after the child is conceived because Yoga can be a superb program for all phases of your life.

72. YOGA IN THE FIRST TRIMESTER

There is no way to avoid it that your body will experience some stunning changes in the primary trimester of your pregnancy. Before that "child knock" ever shows up, you will be extremely mindful that you are experiencing a noteworthy redesign inside your body. When you begin pre-birth Yoga in the main trimester, your educator and you should make sense of what is new with you and modify your Yoga design appropriately. Having an infant isn't care for changing light. It is a remarkable affair for each lady, and your pre-birth Yoga program must mirror your pregnancy and no one else's.

A superior expertise to learn both for your Yoga design and to enable you to adapt to the enormous changes is the means by which to tune in to what is happening inside your body and comprehend it. The influxes of physical and enthusiastic vibes that will experience you in this 12-week time frame will be dramatic to the point that they will overwhelm your core interest. When you take a stake in a customary Yoga program or any physical work out schedule, you take control of your body and instruct it. In the main trimester of pregnancy, as you exploit a pre-birth pregnancy class, you let your body reveal to you what is the correct fit any given day and your Yoga program responds in like manner.

In the 90 days of your first trimester, the opening half a month have their inclination. It is the time when you find that you are pregnant and a large number of the noteworthy manifestations of your pregnancy including the change to your physical shape is still ahead for you. These essential weeks additionally give you an opportunity to influence changes by your Yoga to practice schedule. Try not to be disturbed that you proceeded with your Yoga program in those early weeks as most of the critical changes to your Yoga regimen are imperative later in your pregnancy.

The first trimester is the ideal time to locate a decent pre-birth Yoga program and make that progress. Try not to linger on this progression because before the finish of the main trimester, your physical issues will be a regular concern. Numerous customary Yoga projects, for example, Bikram Yoga are excessively through for you, making it impossible to keep being a piece of when your body turns out to be more delicate and uncommon contemplations should be made for what is happening to you as a result of your pregnancy.

One part of the main trimester that will affect your capacity to be a piece of your Yoga program is morning affliction or general queasiness that can happen to you whenever.

The important advantages of Yoga can fill in as clear motivating force to take up the program at any phase of life. Taking a Yoga class is a standout amongst the best and life avowing things you can do. It is sound, and you get a lot of sweet sentiments from the endorphins that originate from a decent exercise period. Yoga utilises rule that fuses orders of body, psyche and soul so it functions admirably into any intercession or profound projects you may have dynamic in your life. It is amusing to do as such you will end up anticipating Yoga class. That is a significant contrast from different sorts of activity that frequently come up short since you detest them and it's hard to continue going week after week. Yoga class is likewise a social time while having the capacity to work out with companions is a motivation to arrive and stay aware of the program also.

Those advantages are there for you as you start the favoured a very good time as your pregnancy gets in progress. We have talked about the reasonable benefits for pregnant mothers that Yoga can convey also. This is not hypothesis since a large number of pregnant Yoga sweethearts have revealed these benefits. In light of all that, there truly is just a single thing that can impede you beginning investigating pre-birth Yoga. That one thing is a worry about the well-being and medical issues that may originate from being associated with a dynamic action like Yoga.

73. WHAT ARE THE POTENTIAL HEALTH RISKS OF PRENATAL YOGA?

For most ladies who have no referred to well-being worries as you travel through your pregnancy, taking an interest in pre-birth Yoga can have a significant effect in guaranteeing that your pregnancy will bring about a happy and reliable experience for mother and youngster. In any case if you have particular well-being concerns, it is shrewd to consider if Yoga is appropriate for you thoroughly.

Unmistakably the initial step is to counsel with your specialist before beginning any new program, for example, pre-birth Yoga. He or she will have the capacity to guide you or notices about whether your condition is to such an extent that pushing ahead with being a piece of a Yoga program is foolish. While scores of pregnant ladies do in pre-birth Yoga programs if your specialist is not happy with you taking an interest in such a program, dependably mistake to the side of security for you and your newborn child and don't join.

There is now and again a worry that pre-birth Yoga may give you issues in accomplishing the correct adjustments in your weight as you experience your pregnancy. An ideal approach to ensure your weight pick up is solid is to work with your specialist, so your day by day count calories is changed by giving all that you and the child require without over the top weight pick up. When you take an interest in a regular pre-birth Yoga program, it doesn't imply that you will get thinner in an unfortunate way. If anything, the standard exercise will make your digestion consume off undesirable things in your eating regimen and you will keep up a decent eating routine. You may end up eating somewhat more as a result of your activity yet that should just prompt a healthy weight to pick up.

The substantial exercise of pre-birth Yoga exercise will profit your stomach related framework and manufacture muscle gradually and correctly. It will likewise enable you to rest which adds to a substantial weight adjust also. As you encounter more elevated amounts of craving in light of your pre-birth Yoga sessions, take mind that you eat a sound eating regimen that fulfils you and gives substantial sustenance to you and your infant. At that point focus on your weight and converse with your specialist about the perfect weight level for you each phase of your pregnancy. If anything, the Yoga exercise will enable you to keep up a decent eating routine as long as you don't swing to terrible nourishment decisions as a result of your lifted want for sustenance.

A comparable worry that numerous ladies have about going up against pre-birth Yoga is whether Yoga amid pregnancy will help or hurt any circulatory strain issues that they may as of now have. On the off chance that your circulatory strain effects are the consequence of some other restorative condition that puts your pregnancy in a class of one that ought to be observed nearly by your specialist, you should just go up against Yoga if your specialist can see an obvious incentive to you. In any case, a qualified pre-birth Yoga teacher can outline a particular arrangement for Yoga practices that advantage poor course or mulls over exceptional needs and still gives you profits by the breathing and exercise exercises you will gain from a Yoga encounter.

Pre-birth Yoga affects course which helps pulse, processing and disposal. By bringing down the strain in the joints and muscles, Yoga enhances the lymph liquids and general course. Since the course is tolled because of the expanded exercise, the heart and veins work better also.

Over those remarkable medical advantages, pre-birth Yoga builds the versatility of regions of muscle working and also the power and adaptability of joints and muscles. It makes you feel calmer from the back to front which enables stance and decreases to weight on the lower back and knees. These are zones that mothers to-be regularly experience difficulty with so by advancing beyond those issues through Yoga, you take control of your pregnancy in ways that were unrealistic.

74. WOULD IT BE ADVISABLE FOR YOU TO MAKE MODIFICATIONS TO YOUR CURRENT YOGA PLAN DURING PREGNANCY?

The well-being and security contemplations of offering the many advantages of a Yoga program to expecting moms result in the Yoga program getting to be tweaked to the necessities of ladies whose bodies experience dramatic change over the span of nine months. A considerable lot of the Yoga stances and activities are modified given that which is the reason particular Yoga postures are contraindicated amid pregnancy. It is likewise why pre-birth Yoga is best done in an engaged class that is just for mothers to-be and their birthing accomplices or mentors. It is proper for birthing accessories or mentors to be a piece of pre-birth Yoga so they can comprehend the correct approach to utilise Yoga breathing and extending stances to help improve pregnancy and work go.

The facilities that pre-birth Yoga makes when stances or activities are contraindicated amid pregnancy are done to think about the developing waste and to be watchful that the uterus is not packed amid Yoga. This issue is not a major problem amid the first trimester because the uterus is protected by the pelvis and it is still genuinely little. Toward the finish of the first quarter and moving into the second and third quarters, your body will extend drastically, and just the mother to-be will be completely in contact with the amount you have to alter your Yoga program to stay away from uneasiness.

The convenience of the Yoga program amid pre-birth Yoga is not a straightforward thing. It is driven by the necessities of every individual pregnant Yoga class part which puts the obligation on you to be in contact with your body to know when and how much different Yoga postures might be causing you issues. Pregnancy is not time to be gallant or extreme about your exercise plan. On the off chance that you feel uneasiness, whine like there's no tomorrow. Ensuring you can keep on getting the advantages of a tweaked Yoga program without causing you more anxiety and issues than your body is now encountering is the whole motivation behind a pre-birth Yoga program.

Another reason that Yoga practices are contraindicated amid pregnancy originate from the numerous hormonal changes going ahead inside your body as your pregnancy propels. Your body will deliver a particular hormone known as relaxing which is one of nature's methods for altering your tendons and bones with the goal that a child can fit within you. Relaxing diminishes those generally firm internal workings however that makes them more defenseless against getting to be plainly extended amid the months that you are conveying your child. Your pre-birth Yoga mentor will show you how to perceive and maintain a strategic distance from Yoga postures could push you too far and put weight on diminished tendons which could harm them.

As your pregnancy progresses, exceptional accentuation will be put on your knees. Postures will be contraindicated amid pregnancy with the goal that diminished tendons are not extended or harmed in view of Yoga practices that would not be a worry were you not pregnant. In the meantime, you will learn new stances and strategies to keep your knees nimble and solid so you can actually convey that child for nine months and see your knees come back to full adaptability and quality after the birth has happened.

75. YOGA EXERCISES YOU SHOULD NOT DO DURING PREGNANCY

Your specialist and your pre-birth Yoga educator will be as much keener on showing you what not to do as they are about how to utilize great Yoga strategies to profit your pregnancy. This is one of the huge reasons why it is shrewd to change from customary Yoga classes to a pre-birth class when you feel prepared for that progress in your pregnancy. That switch ought to occur when you enter your second trimester.

On the off chance that you are new to Yoga and your classes in pre-birth Yoga are your first introduction to this astonishing control, you have to a lesser extent an issue realising what not to do. Your pre-birth Yoga mentor will deliberately manage you in how to tune into your body and what sorts of stances and activities to keep away from. Be that as it may, there various necessary movements and postures utilised as a part of standard Yoga that ought to be "unlearned" as you move from first to the third trimester in your pre-birth Yoga class. Your eager demeanour about gaining noteworthy ground toward more unpredictable Yoga activities ought to be supplanted totally by a state of mind of learning straightforward and sensible Yoga techniques that will profit you as your pregnancy propels. A portion of the Yoga abilities and strategies to unlearn in pre-birth yoga incorporate...

The general Yoga exercise of playing out a reversal is hazardous because it could make you fall toward the divider which is risky for mother and unborn tyke.

CONCLUSION

Thank you for downloading this book I hope you will apply the acquired knowledge productively. Having a sound pregnancy begins with setting up your body for this mind blowing cycle of pregnancy some time before you wind up noticeably pregnant. An inadequate egg or sperm has an enormous part to play with regards to the motivation behind why such a large number of ladies lose. Deficient eggs or sperms are regularly because of inadequate vitamins, minerals and cancer prevention agents in the body. Solid pregnancy arrangement will diminish your danger of intrinsic irregularities, unnatural birth cycles and going into untimely work. Pregnancy is much more than a physical procedure that happens to a lady. It has a mind boggling mental, enthusiastic, profound and vigorous side to it. Keeping in mind the end goal to have a solid pregnancy you should grasp pregnancy from an all-encompassing body, brain and soul.